65 Answers

about Psychiatric Conditions

RICHA BHATIA, MD

DISCLAIMERS AND AUTHOR'S NOTE

The contents of this book are for informational purposes only. The author does not warrant that the information contained in this book is complete and accurate. Each of the fields of medicine and psychiatry are a delicate amalgamation of science and art, and their inherent complexity makes it unfeasible to explain in detail every nuance or exception that may relate to any topic. Even the simplest question and answer would require years of medical education and professional experience before it could be applied to a 'real life' situation. In no way, should any content of this book be construed as medical or psychiatric advice or recommendations, or as diagnostic or treatment opinion for any medical or psychiatric disorder. You should seek the consultation of a licensed physician or health care professional, if you suspect that you or a family member is suffering from a psychiatric or a medical condition. If in any medical or psychiatric crisis or if you or someone you know is struggling, please call 911 or go (or take the individual) to the nearest emergency room immediately.

The author and publisher expressly disclaim liability for any adverse effects arising from the use or application of information contained in this book. Under no circumstances, will any legal responsibility, liability or blame be held against the author or publisher for any damages, loss or reparation due to the information herein, either directly or indirectly. The reader assumes sole and utter responsibility and risk.

Portions of this book have been taken from the author's book: 'Demystifying Psychiatric Conditions and Treatments: And Answers to Your Commonly Asked Questions', published in 2018.

The author has no financial conflicts of interest with any products, brands/manufacturers, or devices mentioned in this book.

It is worth noting that there are many research findings that are well-known and frequently cited in psychiatry. The author has done her best to reference any findings where the source is known. The author extends her apologies to the originators of any findings, who may have been unintentionally overlooked.

Each of the questions in this book is a hypothetical scenario that the author has invented, along with invented traits and features- none of the questions or content of this book represent an actual or real patient.

Opinions or views expressed in this book are those of the author, and do not represent the opinions or views of any institutions or organizations the author has been affiliated with.

Table of Contents

ACKNOWLEDGEMENTS

This book draws on existing scientific evidence in the field of psychiatry as well as from my own experience treating individuals suffering from various psychiatric conditions. The available evidence in psychiatry is a product of the work of many physicians, scientists and researchers over the years.

I have had the privilege to see a few thousand patients of all age groups, either directly or indirectly by supervising residents and fellows. This book is dedicated to all these individuals and to millions of others suffering from mental health disorders, with the hope that more and more people gain awareness about psychiatric disorders and treatments. Awareness about psychiatric disorders is a necessity, not a luxury.

I owe many thanks to my mentors who have been a constant source of inspiration over the years. Finally, many thanks to my family – Nimish, Sushil, Hirdesh, Divya, for their unconditional support and encouragement.

INTRODUCTION

Mental health is an integral part of overall health and well-being. Psychiatric disorders have been proven to have a biological basis (in addition to psychological underpinnings). The consequences of not getting treatment for psychiatric disorders can be many, and at times, severe. This book aims to answer some questions about psychiatric disorders and treatments, with the goal to decrease stigma and enhance awareness about psychiatric disorders and treatments. This has been written in an easy to understand question and answer format.

You may notice that I often mention the word 'options' in my book. This is because there are different options among psychiatric treatments. What works for one person may be different from what works for another, depending on the medical history, family history, various symptoms, and other factors. There is no 'one size fits all' in psychiatry or medicine. A certain set of symptoms may have several diagnostic possibilities. Many factors and intricate nuances go into determining the right diagnosis and suitable treatment options. It is important to consult a physician or a specialist and to bring forth your concerns with them in detail.

Again, this book is not intended to give any sort of advice or diagnostic opinion or recommendation and must not be construed in this way. The goal of this book is solely to raise awareness. The questions and answers in this book are hypothetical, invented examples and not real-life answers or advice. The contents of this book aim to shed light on some of the disorders, possibilities and options in psychiatry and are by no means exhaustive and are not a complete review of the subject. Only a psychiatrist or physician who has examined you can advise you about your condition, diagnosis and/or treatment.

Depression

Depression is a common psychiatric condition. It is estimated by the World Health Organization that about 300 million people suffer from depression worldwide.

Depression can be a debilitating disorder. Functional MRI studies of the brain show changes in brains of depressed individuals. The good news is that effective treatments for depression are available, and the hope is that more and more people seek treatment rather than suffering silently. Each of the following examples of questions and answers is hypothetical. The goal of these is to improve awareness about depression, reduce stigma and help the reader better understand some aspects of depressive disorders and treatment options.

1. What is postpartum depression? Is there treatment for it? How is it different from 'baby blues'?

Postpartum depression is more than the 'baby blues' that many mothers experience after the birth of a child. Baby blues are characterized by crying spells, mood swings, and anxiety. On the other hand, women with postpartum depression may experience feelings of hopelessness, excessive guilt or worthlessness, loss of interest in pleasurable activities, thoughts of suicide, or even thoughts of hurting the baby, in addition to other depressive symptoms. Mood changes in postpartum depression tend to be more pervasive and significant than those in baby blues.

Postpartum depression is not uncommon. It is a serious condition, posing risks to both the mother and the infant, if untreated. Therefore, it warrants treatment and timely assessment by a licensed mental health clinician.

Women at higher risk for postpartum depression are those with a prior history of depression, family history of depression, a medically complicated pregnancy or delivery, lack of spousal or social support, and presence of other stressors during pregnancy.

Treatment for postpartum depression can be through psychotherapy and/or medications. Your doctor will advise you about breastfeeding options, if you take an antidepressant medication during this period. Certain antidepressants have been shown to be secreted in lesser amounts in breast milk as compared to others. Those are therefore, considered safer if you plan to breastfeed.

Social, family support is obviously a key factor that can help the mother recover optimally.

Talk to your doctor if you or a friend/family member observe or experience any of these concerns.

2. Why Treat Depression?

Studies show that major depressive disorder is a risk factor for some serious health conditions, such as coronary artery disease, diabetes, stroke and even some cancers.

Having untreated depression on top of a medical condition (such as diabetes, heart disease or other) usually means that the course of the medical condition may get worse than usual. Treatment is key.

fMRI brain studies of depressed individuals show that untreated depression can cause structural brain changes. In addition, physiological changes in the body (for example, changes in stress hormone, cortisol) occur as a result of untreated depression. Untreated depression increases the likelihood that depressive episodes may become more severe and pervasive or unremitting over time. Untreated depression poses the risk of suicide. Suicide is the second leading cause of death among 15-34 year olds, according to a 2015 report by the Centers for Disease Control and Prevention (CDC). The National Suicide Prevention Lifeline (for USA) is confidential and available 24 hours a day, 7 days a week at 1-800-273-8255. You can also text at the 24x7 Crisis Text Line (Text HOME to 741741 in the US). International hotlines can be found on the website suicide.org

Seeking timely help from a physician/mental health professional can make a huge difference. In addition, family and friends can help a depressed individual in many ways- such as, by non-judgemental support, availability and by helping the individual seek professional help.

3. What is depression?

Depression is a clinical term. It differs from 'sadness' which is a normal human emotion that everyone experiences at times. Clinical depression is characterized by pervasive or significant sad or low mood that continues over a certain period of time. In addition, it is accompanied by at least a few other symptoms, such as loss of interest in pleasurable activities, low energy, poor concentration, worthlessness, hopelessness, changes in sleep or appetite, and/or suicidal thoughts. You don't have to have all of the above symptoms to meet the criteria of a depressive disorder.

Depression is a common and treatable condition. There are several treatment options for depression. Early recognition and timely treatment is important.

4. How common is Depression? Who can it affect?

Depression has a high prevalence. According to the World Health Organization, 'depression is the leading cause of ill health and disability worldwide' and it is estimated that 'more than 300 million people are now living with depression, an increase of more than 18% between 2005 and 2015' (WHO).

Depression is overall more common in females than males, however, it can affect anyone. Males may be less likely to seek help for depression. Individuals with a family history of depression are more likely to suffer from depression at some point in life. However, having a family history does not mean that one will necessarily suffer from depression.

There are effective treatments available for depression, ranging from psychotherapy (more widely known as 'therapy'), medications, to ECT (Electroconvulsive therapy), TMS (Transcranial Magnetic Stimulation) and others, (depending on the type and severity of depression).

Several different types of psychotherapy options as well as medication options, are available. The most suitable treatment option may differ from person to person, depending on several factors (such as medical history, family history, severity and other characteristics of the depressive episode, any prior treatment options, and other factors).

5. **Can I take an antidepressant just when I feel low, and stop it the next day if I am feeling better?**

An antidepressant usually does not work that way. Consult your doctor for any medication questions- do not make any medication changes on your own. Most medications for depression (SSRIs, SNRIs, TCAs) are taken daily. If one does not take them regularly as prescribed, they are not likely to be effective, as they work by building up in the system over time, as opposed to certain medications such as acetaminophen (brand name 'tylenol') which may start taking effect within an hour. Missed doses of SSRIs (selective serotonin re-uptake inhibitors- a common class of antidepressants used these days) can lead to discontinuation symptoms, such as flu-like symptoms, stomach upset, nausea, vomiting, headache, sleep problems, mood changes, increase in anxiety as well as a likelihood of relapse of depression.

6. My husband 'acts depressed'. I've been asking him to 'be stronger', but, he doesn't seem to get it. If only, he would go out and do things, it would be better. Am I missing something?

If suspecting depression, help your family member consult a physician/ psychiatrist who will do a thorough evaluation to determine the right diagnosis and choice of treatment for your family member. Depression is a disease, which involves the brain. Effective treatment for depression is available.

It is important to treat depression. Brain imaging studies show that treatment for depression can create positive brain changes.

It is important to remember that depression is not a character weakness, as old myths portrayed it to be. Depression has biological (brain based) and psychological underpinnings. fMRI scans of depressed individuals show differences in brain activity from non-depressed individuals. Recent studies show a smaller volume of certain parts of the brain in depressed individuals. Having a family history of depression can make it more likely for one to have depression. However, depression can affect anyone.

Although behavioral activation techniques such as avoiding isolation and exercising can help with depression, assuming that an individual 'can do it' and is just choosing not to do things or is being 'lazy', is a mistaken and risky assumption.

Depressive disorders require treatment. Treatment can be in the form of medications and/or psychotherapy. Occasionally, ECT (electroconvulsive therapy) or TMS (Transcranial Magnetic Stimulation) may be offered and utilized for severe depression.

Which treatment option is most appropriate in a certain situation is usually a collaborative decision between a patient and their physician. One should be forthcoming with their physician so that the most suitable treatment option can be found.

Untreated depression poses the risk of future prolonged and worsening episodes of depression, in addition to risk of suicide and worsening physical health, therefore, treatment should be sought in a timely manner. Also, it is important to rule out any medical conditions which could be mimicking depression. Hypothyroidism, brain masses, even certain cancers can manifest in the form of depression.

Just the way it is important to get treatment for diabetes or heart disease, similarly, it is also important to get treatment for depression. Treatment can be life-saving.

7. Do Children Get Depressed?

Yes, children and teens can suffer from depression. Psychiatrists/pediatricians can assess for, diagnose and treat childhood depression.

Depression in children manifests more often in the form of irritability or even anger. Decline in school functioning, especially if it is new or recent onset, may occur due to depression. Social withdrawal, decreased interest in fun activities, talking about dying, death or suicide, rejection hypersensitivity, frequent pains and aches, running away from home or talking about it, changes in energy, sleep or appetite, are some of the signs of depression in children.

According to the Centers for Disease Control and Prevention (CDC) report, suicide was the third leading cause of death among ages 10-14 in the United States in 2015. It is very important to identify and treat depression in childhood and adolescence. Untreated childhood depression can increase risk of prolonged, more severe episodes of depression over time, besides causing poor functioning and posing risk of suicide.

Effective treatment options have been widely researched and are available for childhood depression. Timely recognition and treatment is key.

8. What is the treatment for depression in children and teens?

If suspecting that your child or teen is suffering from depression, talk to your child's doctor for a complete evaluation and to discuss treatment options.
In general, according to current evidence, psychotherapy is the treatment of choice for children and adolescents with mild to moderate depression. Cognitive behavioral therapy (CBT) may be used for children older than age 11. For younger children- behavioral therapy, child directed play therapy, psychodynamic psychotherapy may be the kinds of psychotherapies utilized, depending on the age, the psychological mindedness of the child/teen, and the nature of the depressive condition.

A combination of CBT and SSRI (Selective Serotonin Re-Uptake Inhibitors) medications is the treatment of choice for moderate to severe depression in children and adolescents.

Other treatment options may be utilized in certain situations.

If childhood depression is treated in a timely manner, the likelihood of relapse and future worsening is significantly lesser.

9. **My mom is in her 80s. A year ago, she had a heart attack. She doesn't seem interested in anything anymore, which is unlike her. She's probably just feeling lonely. Do I do something about it?**

Talk to your mother, and her physician to get her evaluated comprehensively.

In general, in addition to a thorough medical evaluation by a physician, assessment for depression by a physician is important in the elderly, as depression in elderly people is common. However, depression in elderly is often under-diagnosed or missed, mostly due to lack of awareness and other factors. Depression after a heart attack is common.

Depression is especially more likely when there are accompanying medical conditions, such as heart disease, stroke or cancer, that are impairing functioning or causing disability.

The good news is that depression in older adults is treatable, often with psychotherapy, medications or both. SSRIs (Selective serotonin reuptake inhibitors) are often used for depression after myocardial infarction. Certain SSRIs have been tested widely for use after a heart attack, with good benefit. A doctor will review the entire medical history and determine which SSRI/antidepressant (if needed)/other treatment option may be most suitable.

Social support and preventing isolation are additional key factors in reducing the likelihood of depression after a heart attack.

10. How to know which antidepressant medication is best for me?

Your physician will help you find the most suitable option for your condition.

In general, the choice of an antidepressant medication depends on one's specific symptoms (for example, someone who is feeling lethargic may benefit from an activating antidepressant such as bupropion; on the other hand, an underweight individual who is not sleeping well may require a sedating, appetite promoting antidepressant such as mirtazapine).

A complete evaluation by a physician is important as many factors and details involving one's family history, psychological, biological and other history go into making such a decision.

For example, factors that influence the choice of antidepressant are one's medical history (for instance, certain medications are considered safer in individuals with a history of cardiac disease), prior medication trials, one's family history of response to antidepressants (evidence shows that if your immediate family member benefitted from a certain SSRI, you may have a higher likelihood of responding well to it), and other factors such as potential interactions with other medications one might be taking.

11. I plan to get pregnant in the next year or so. I think I should stop my antidepressant now.

The decision to continue psychotropic medications or not during pregnancy is not a simple one. In general, if one plans to get pregnant in the near future, it is important to consult the prescribing doctor on a regular basis to collaboratively make a decision about continuing psychotropic medications or not. Your prescribing doctor and you are best familiar with how your psychiatric condition has been.

The prescribing doctor will do a comprehensive evaluation of risks and benefits of continuing a particular medication during pregnancy versus risks of the untreated psychiatric condition to you and the baby, to collaboratively determine the most suitable course of action. It is important to note that different medications pose different levels of risks during pregnancy. For example, certain medications such as benzodiazepines, paroxetine pose more risks to the fetus than does fluoxetine. Also, certain times during the gestational period are safer for use of medications than others. In general, it may be advisable to exercise caution with use of psychotropic medications during pregnancy, especially if the psychiatric condition is mild to moderate. However, untreated depression, bipolar disorder or schizophrenia can also pose serious risks to mothers as well as to babies (including, but not limited to, worsening of the mother's psychiatric condition, resulting safety risks to mother and/baby, risk of preterm labor, low birth weight, etc.). All these factors are taken into account while making this decision. If pregnant, psychotherapy can also be a beneficial treatment option for many psychiatric conditions.

In summary, this is not a decision one should be making by oneself. If a change in dosage, or switching to a different, safer medication, or discontinuation of a medication is required, the prescribing doctor can help one do so.

For further reading, see the following link from Massachusetts General Hospital, regarding use of psychotropic medications during pregnancy and breastfeeding:

https://womensmentalhealth.org/specialty-clinics/psychiatric-disorders-during-pregnancy/

12. **I am afraid to mention the word 'suicide' to my sister who is depressed. I am worried about her, but, I think asking about suicide might make her have suicidal thoughts. Is that true?**

In general, asking about suicidal thoughts does not make one suicidal. If you or someone you know is feeling suicidal, it is an emergency. Seeking immediate help is of prime importance. Go (or take the individual) to the nearest emergency room or call 911.

Following are some suicide help resources:

National Suicide Prevention Lifeline: **1–800–273–TALK (8255)**, confidential, 24x7. www.suicidepreventionlifeline.org

Crisis Text Line: text START to 741–741

Someone who is struggling with depression may already have contemplated or thought about suicide, without others knowing. Maybe, they are afraid to talk about it or mention it for various reasons. Knowing that depression is a treatable disease, and that help, support and effective treatment are available, is important.

If you are concerned about someone suffering from depression, support them and urge them to seek the help of a psychiatrist or a therapist or a physician. Having social support and meaningful connections can make a significant difference, in addition to treatment. Just the way it is important to get treatment for diabetes or heart disease, similarly, it is important to get treatment for depression. Treatment can be life-saving.

13. My friend whose husband died a year ago, has been making comments that she wants to die as well. She frequently says she has nothing to look forward to, and has withdrawn from most activities. Is this normal after the death of a loved one?

If you or someone you know is feeling suicidal, it is an emergency. Seeking immediate help is of prime importance. Go (or take the individual) to the nearest emergency room or call 911.

Grief is different from clinical depression. A psychiatrist or a psychologist would be able to help differentiate between normal grief versus a major depressive disorder, after examining the affected person.

A grief reaction involves sad mood, missing the loved one or intense longing for the loved one. On the other hand, having suicidal thoughts, frequent feelings of hopelessness or extreme worthlessness are usually signs of a major depressive order rather than a grief reaction.

There are grief support groups that can help the grieving person mourn and process the loss of a loved one.

On the other hand, if one is concerned about a friend or a family member suffering from depression after the death of a loved one, support them, educate them about it and urge them to seek the help of a psychiatrist or a therapist for treatment.

The following are some suicide help resources:

National Suicide Prevention Lifeline: 1–800–273–TALK (8255), confidential, 24x7. www.suicidepreventionlifeline.org

Crisis Text Line: text START to 741–741

14. X medication worked great for depression for my friend. I think I am depressed; I should try it too.

It is important to ask your doctor about various medication and other treatment options available for your condition, so that you can make an informed choice, suitable for your specific condition. There are various effective, beneficial treatments available for depression.

Different individuals may respond differently to the same medication, so, a medication that worked great for your friend may or may not work as well for you.

Do not assume what your diagnosis is, without consulting a physician or a specialist. Discuss your concerns with your doctor in detail; they should be able to provide you with an accurate diagnosis after doing an assessment.

15. My doctor prescribed me citalopram (brand name, 'Celexa') for depression. I went to the pharmacy to pick it up and came across St John's wort in the aisle. I think I should take that too, since I've read it can help depression. I know my doctor is not a naturopath, so, I guess I don't need to tell him about it?

Do tell your doctor right away about any herbal or other treatments you might be taking or intend to take. Even herbal remedies often interact with psychotropic medications. Your doctor has the knowledge of interactions that this herbal remedy may cause, when combined with citalopram (SSRI), and will advise you about those.

In general, St John's wort is known to be a serotonergic agent. This means, when taken in combination with another serotonergic agent such as citalopram, it can increase the likelihood that one will end up with too much serotonin in the body. This may manifest in the form of milder problems, such as tremors, stomach upset, activation, but, occasionally, can lead to a full-blown serotonin syndrome which can be life-threatening and warrants emergency medical attention. In addition, St John's wort can cause similar interactions with other antidepressants (older antidepressants such as TCAs-amitriptyline, imipramine, MAO Inhibitors such as selegiline), and even with cough medications and certain migraine medications. In general, St John's wort should not be used with any antidepressant.

Talk to your doctor for recommendations specific to your situation.

16. I feel very sad during the winter months. It gets better when spring starts. This has been happening for the last 3 winters. I lose energy, interest and motivation for any fun activities during the winters. What might this be, and what might help?

Consulting a physician for a complete evaluation, diagnosis and treatment is important.

In general, depressive symptoms (such as sad or low mood, loss of interest, low energy, changes in sleep, appetite, low concentration) that occur only during the winters and resolve by spring, fall under the category of seasonal affective disorder.
Bright light treatment for about 30 minutes a day every morning can be helpful. Some people may need antidepressant and/or psychotherapy treatment in addition.

It is important to buy the appropriate lightbox designed specifically for seasonal affective disorder (or seasonal depression). Your physician can guide you towards the kind and intensity of lightbox treatment most suitable for you.

In general, a lightbox used for this purpose should emit the least amount of ultraviolet light, and you should keep your eyes away from it to avoid any UV damage to eyes.

Also, many people living in cold climates and/or during winter months develop Vitamin D deficiency. Low vitamin D is linked with depression and fatigue (in addition to increasing risk for heart disease, hypothyroidism, osteoporosis).

Although Vitamin D alone is not adequate for treatment of depression, it is worthwhile to get your Vitamin D levels checked, and supplement if needed.

Vitamin D supplementation can reverse the vitamin D deficit. A vitamin D level between 40 to 60 is optimal.

17. **My doctor advised me to get ECT treatment. I suffer from severe depression and have tried many medications. Nothing has worked much so far. But, I am afraid about ECT as I've heard so much about it. I saw in a movie that it is dangerous.**

Discuss your concerns with your psychiatrist so that you can make an informed decision whether ECT is an appropriate and suitable choice for treatment of your condition.

In general, despite strong research evidence showing efficacy of ECT, there is still myth surrounding ECT (Electroconvulsive Therapy). Some of this may be due to how it was portrayed in old movies, such as One Flew Over the Cuckoo's Nest. In present times, ECT is performed vastly differently than how it was shown in that movie. Nowadays, ECT is done under general anesthesia. Similar to any procedure done under general anesthesia, the risks from general anesthesia are there, but, ECT has been proven to be safe and effective for severe, treatment resistant depression and suicidal thoughts, even for pregnant women.

In special circumstances, such as if you had a heart attack recently, or a certain kind of brain mass or stroke, you will need specialized assessment by a cardiologist and/or a neurologist to determine if ECT is safe for you. But, there is no absolute contraindication for ECT. Even if you don't have any medical condition, you will be assessed by an anesthesiologist (in addition to your psychiatrist) and undergo tests such as an EKG, lab testing, and in some cases, a brain CT or an MRI scan, before you are deemed to be a suitable candidate for ECT.

The good news is that ECT can be very effective for severe depression and starts working quicker than most antidepressant medications.

18. I have been suffering from severe depression for many years. None of the medications I have tried have worked. Are there any other treatment options besides medications and therapy?

Consult your physician/psychiatrist for treatment options for your depression, to find one most suitable for you. A complete medical assessment can rule out any underlying medical conditions that may be causing depression.

In general, there are genetic tests available that can identify the antidepressant medications that are more likely to work for you. ECT (Electroconvulsive therapy) and TMS (Transcranial Magnetic Stimulation) are some other treatment options for severe depression. Both have been widely used and researched, and have been found to be overall safe and effective.

I have treated hundreds of patients with ECT with positive outcomes. A large percentage of patients with severe depression experience a dramatic improvement with ECT.

ECT these days is performed under general anesthesia. The vast majority of people undergoing ECT do not experience any permanent or irreversible side effects. Common side effects from ECT are headaches (lasting up to a few hours), drowsiness or sleepiness, short-term memory loss (typically reversible). It is worthwhile noting that not everyone experiences these side effects. Rare, but, more serious risks could be those related to general anesthesia and cardiac complications. An anesthesia and cardiac assessment serves to determine if one is a suitable candidate for ECT.

ECT is performed in a course of 8-12 treatments, often starting with 3 treatments a week. Some people may require maintenance ECT treatment after completion of the initial course, depending on the severity of depression.

TMS (or Transcranial Magnetic Stimulation) is newer than ECT. It has been shown to work well for severe depression. TMS does not require general anesthesia, so, side effects are even lesser as compared to ECT. Headaches, muscle aches can be some of the possible side effects. Patients can usually drive themselves home after a TMS session.

Other, newer treatment options, such as ketamine, vagal nerve stimulation, are being researched for treatment of severe depression as well. Ketamine has been shown to have a dramatic response in severe depression, at least during the initial period. Ketamine treatment is being offered at various clinics.

19. **My child is making comments like 'I don't care whether I live or die'. I don't think he knows much about life or death. He may have just heard someone saying it, right?**

Call 911 or take your child/teen to the nearest emergency room if they are experiencing suicidal thoughts/death wishes/thoughts of hurting self.
If noticing any recent changes in mood, behavior or functioning of your child, consult your child's pediatrician/psychiatrist for evaluation and treatment. (Get a referral for a psychiatrist if needed)

Following are some suicide help resources:

National Suicide Prevention Lifeline: **1–800–273–TALK (8255)**, confidential, 24x7. www.suicidepreventionlifeline.org

Crisis Text Line: text START to 741–741

Thoughts or comments about death should be taken seriously, regardless of the age of the person making such a comment. Writing goodbye letters, giving away beloved possessions, talking about plans to end life, are additional serious signs of suicidality.

Young children, especially under age 7, may not understand the finality or irreversibility of death, but, may still experience suicidal thoughts. Given higher level of impulsivity among children and teens as compared to adults, they may even be at a higher risk of acting on suicidal thoughts. There are effective treatments for depression and suicidal thoughts in children and teens. An evaluation by a psychiatrist/pediatrician is an important step to get your child the necessary treatment.

20. What are the different types of antidepressants?

Antidepressant medications belong to mainly 3 categories: SSRIs (selective serotonin re-uptake inhibitors), SNRIs (serotonin and norepinephrine re-uptake inhibitors), and TCAs (Tricyclic Antidepressants or older antidepressants). SSRIs and SNRIs are newer than Tricyclic antidepressants, and in general, have a lower side effect profile than TCAs.

All these classes of antidepressants have been proven to be effective, according to substantial research evidence. In addition, another class of medications is MAO Inhibitors which are less commonly used nowadays. MAO Inhibitors, although effective for certain kinds of depression, require stringent monitoring of diet, due to risk of potentially life-threatening hypertensive crisis when combined with certain foods.

One of the most commonly used MAO Inhibitors is selegiline.

There are other antidepressants which do not belong to the above-mentioned categories, such as Mirtazapine (known by brand name, Remeron) which is mainly serotonergic but, works differently than an SSRI; Bupropion (known by brand name, Wellbutrin) which acts on dopamine and norepinephrine, improves energy, lowers appetite, but, may increase anxiety in the short term. Newer antidepressants are worth mentioning, such as vortioxetine (also known by brand name, Trintellix) which acts on serotonin receptors in the brain and is used for depression.

21. What are the different SSRIs, and how long do they take to work?

SSRIs (Selective Serotonin Re-Uptake Inhibitors) have been the most commonly used antidepressants in recent years. SSRIs include fluoxetine (also known by brand name, Prozac), sertraline (also known by brand name, Zoloft), escitalopram (also known by brand name, Lexapro), paroxetine (also known by brand name, Paxil), citalopram (also known by brand name, Celexa), fluvoxamine (also known by brand name, Luvox), vilazodone (brand name, Vibryd).
Serotonin is a neurochemical, the alterations of which are implicated in the pathophysiology of depression. SSRIs work by making the neurochemical serotonin more available in the brain.

SSRIs take effect over time-they do not start working right away. Most studies show that they can take 4-6 weeks to start working, and up to 12 weeks for a full effect. However, some individuals may start experiencing benefits as early as 2-3 weeks from the time of initiation.

22. Is there an SSRI that is better for depression than others?

After examining you and evaluating your complete history, your doctor will be able to advise you on the treatment option or medication most suitable for you.

In general, studies show that most SSRIs are comparable in terms of efficacy for depression. However, different individuals may respond differently to the same SSRI.

All SSRIs are FDA approved for depression in adults, except for fluvoxamine (which is used more commonly for Obsessive Compulsive Disorder). If you have an immediate family member who responded well to a certain antidepressant, you may have a higher likelihood of responding well to the same antidepressant (however, this is not necessary).

23. What are the Side Effects of SSRIs?

Common initial side effects may be headaches or GI side effects (stomach upset, nausea, vomiting). For most people, these tend to resolve within the first few days of starting medication. Other potential side effects are sleepiness/sedation, potential increase in weight (most studies do not show a weight gain of >3-4 lbs a year with SSRIs), increased risk of bleeding (tell your psychiatrist if you have a bleeding disorder or other related condition, and/or if you have a surgical procedure coming up), sexual side effects (delayed ejaculation, possible decreased libido), activation/increase in anxiety (especially common with faster dose increase), precipitation of mania or hypomania in predisposed individuals.

Refer to the manufacturer's medication pamphlet for a complete, exhaustive list of possible side effects.

Note: Any medication can cause an allergic reaction or a rash. If you notice a new rash with the start or increase in dose of any medication, consult your doctor immediately. Your doctor may ask you to stop the medication and will make further recommendations based on rash condition and severity. If you notice an allergic reaction, consult your doctor immediately who will advise you on the next steps. For any severe side effects, go to the emergency room.

Not everyone taking a certain psychotropic medication will have side effects. Many people experience no known side effects when taking antidepressants.

ADHD

ADHD (or Attention Deficit Hyperactivity Disorder) is a condition which involves difficulty with attention, hyperactivity and/or impulsivity. One does not need to have all of these three categories of symptoms to have ADHD. ADHD, when untreated, can affect school or work performance, increase risk of substance use, motor vehicle accidents and other difficulties. Effective treatment is available for ADHD. It is important to rule out any medical or other psychiatric condition before arriving to this diagnosis, as causes of inattention can be many.

24. My child has ADHD. His pediatrician wants him to take ADHD medications. His ADHD is bad, but, I am thinking of trying fish oil instead. Also, it might work if I urge him to study more. What do you think?

Depending on your child's medical history and the severity of ADHD, various medication and treatment options can be explored with your doctor to find the most suitable fit that is also safe and well-tolerated.

ADHD or Attention deficit Hyperactivity disorder is one of those psychiatric conditions which have been proven to have a clear biological basis. In simple terms, you can think of this biological basis as an anomaly in the neuronal wiring in the frontal lobe of the brain. Because the underlying basis has been shown to be strongly biological (based on research so far), evidence-based guidelines suggest that medications are the cornerstone of ADHD treatment, particularly for ADHD that is moderate to severe.

Stimulant based ADHD medications work by modulating the dopamine balance in the frontal lobe of the brain. Norepinephrine is another neurochemical associated with attention. Non-stimulant medications for ADHD, such as atomoxetine, act via modulating primarily norepinephrine along with other neurotransmitters.

In general, fish oil has not been shown to have conclusive evidence for treatment of ADHD, and it is not FDA approved. Some studies have shown some small benefit with use of fish oil, others have not shown significant benefit as compared to ADHD medications. If you would like to use fish oil, ask your child's pediatrician first to ensure that adding it does not pose any risks to any medical conditions or medications your child may have.

Based on what we know so far, unlike psychotherapy for depression and anxiety, psychotherapy for ADHD does not modify the brain wiring responsible for hyperactivity, inattention or impulsivity in ADHD. However, it can certainly help with organizational strategies to manage ADHD, and in the case of children with ADHD, psychotherapy based interventions such as parent behavior modification training can be very helpful as an adjunct. Psychotherapy can also be beneficial for any anxiety and depressive symptoms associated with or secondary to the sequelae of untreated ADHD.

Urging your child to study harder is not likely to result in resolution of the difficulty focusing.

Interventions that can be helpful at school and at home, are:

- 1:1 attention while doing schoolwork/homework,

- shorter assignments,
- brief breaks built in that allow the child/teen to get up and engage in some physical activity,
- a higher ratio of positive to constructive feedback,
- assistance with schedules and reminders,
- Occasionally, a timer for completing each small section of a task can be helpful.

Some latest research is also exploring neurofeedback as an option to treat ADHD.

25. My son's ADHD medication does not let him sleep. What can I do?

Consult your child's prescribing physician to discuss options and the next best course of action suitable to your situation.

Stimulant based ADHD medications (methylphenidate or amphetamine- based formulations) can cause difficulty falling asleep.

In general, there can be a few, different options to manage this, depending on the specific situation, history and other factors:

- Move timing of medication to a time earlier in the day when possible
- Reduce dose of medication if feasible
- Combine with low dose of a non-stimulant ADHD medication, such as guanfacine or clonidine which

have sedating properties (as long as medical history allows)

- Practice sleep hygiene measures (avoid electronics prior to bedtime, avoid bright lights prior to bedtime, have a regular bedtime, use bed only for sleep, ensure comfortable temperature in the room, avoid physical activity too late in the day)
- If none of these is effective, switching to a different medication (a different stimulant medication, or a non-stimulant medication such as atomoxetine) is an option

Each individual's symptoms, severity, and medical history are different, and warrant a careful consideration of the various factors, to come to an informed decision. This is what a psychiatrist specializes in. What's suitable for one individual may not be appropriate/suitable for another.

26. I don't want my child to take stimulant medications for ADHD. Are there other medication options besides stimulants?

Talk to your child's pediatrician about the most suitable ADHD medication option for your child.

Yes, there are non-stimulant medications as well. These include medications such as clonidine and guanfacine, and their longer acting versions known by the brand names of Kapvay and Intuniv respectively.

Other non-stimulant medications for ADHD include atomoxetine (also known by brand name, Strattera).

These medicines work by acting on different receptors in the brain than stimulant medications. Clonidine, guanfacine or atomoxetine are not controlled substances, and do not pose risk of dependence.

Clonidine and guanfacine do not cause appetite suppression, weight loss, tic exacerbation, increase in blood pressure, or difficulty falling asleep, all of which are potential side effects and risks with stimulant medications.

On the other hand, clonidine and guanfacine may actually help tics, insomnia, and may cause lowering of blood pressure (and therefore, require regular blood pressure monitoring by the physician). Due to lowering of blood pressure, some people may experience lightheadedness/dizziness or drowsiness with these medications. This effect may be more prominent with clonidine than with guanfacine.

Clonidine and guanfacine tend to address hyperactivity and impulsivity more than they address inattention.

The most suitable medication option may depend on several different factors, such as the medical history of the individual, body weight, tolerability of medication, family history of response to a particular medication, severity of the disorder, prior medication trials and response to them, and other factors.

27. I went online and diagnosed myself with ADHD; I want my doctor to prescribe me 'Ritalin' for it. He's not agreeing with me; what should I do?

It can be risky to diagnose yourself. You are not equipped with the intricate nuances of medical knowledge to do so. If you suspect you have a psychiatric or medical condition, you must bring these concerns up with your doctor. A licensed physician or psychologist can make a psychiatric diagnosis. After a comprehensive evaluation, your doctor will discuss their clinical impressions with you.

Psychotropic medications, especially 'ritalin', are serious business. Whether taking a psychotropic medication is going to be safe and recommended for you, can only be determined by your doctor.

Do not pressure your doctor to prescribe a certain medication. If they are saying no to a certain medication, there is usually a clinical rationale behind it. Your doctor went to school for several years to be able to prescribe properly and accurately. Misdiagnosis can mean that you end up taking the wrong medications for a condition you do not have, and in some cases, can be life-threatening if the actual underlying condition is missed and not treated. There have been even reports of sudden deaths of people who misused medications or took them on their own accord.

28. My son likes to eat a lot of sugar. Will this cause ADHD?

A few animal studies have shown increased risk of depression, weakened memory and anxiety with high sugar intake. However, eating too much sugar, while obviously not beneficial for optimal health, is not known to cause ADHD.

The exact causes of ADHD are still being researched. Genetic factors have been implicated in causation, so, having a parent or sibling with ADHD significantly increases risk.

Promoting a healthy and balanced diet for children, in general, is important for better mood, energy and sleep which are all linked with better focusing ability.

If your child is showing signs of inattention, hyperactivity and/or impulsivity on a frequent basis, consult your child's doctor for an assessment.

29.Is it normal to have difficulty focusing? When is difficulty focusing 'ADHD'?

In general, most children, teens or adults suffer from some difficulty focusing or sustaining attention at one time or another in their life. Often, when people are undergoing major life events or multiple stressors, they may experience difficulties focusing or concentrating. ADHD is diagnosed when difficulty focusing, hyperactivity and/or impulsivity starts before age 12, this difficulty is pervasive and significantly impairing school, work, and/or social functioning of an individual, and cannot be explained by another psychiatric or medical condition, according to criteria set by the Diagnostic and Statistical Manual of Psychiatry (DSM-5).

ADHD is both under-diagnosed and over-diagnosed.

The diagnosis of ADHD is often missed, which is unfortunate, given that there are effective treatments for ADHD. On the other hand, sometimes, people assume they have ADHD, without consulting a specialist or an expert. This can have serious repercussions, as the causes of attention difficulties can be several. ADHD is not the only cause.

Assuming the diagnosis as ADHD (or something else) without a thorough assessment from a physician, creates the risk of missing the actual underlying diagnosis and treatment.

30.I have tried good doses of different stimulant and non-stimulant medications for my child, since she started showing attention problems 2 years ago, but, nothing has worked so far. What do I do?

In general, if several, different classes of medications for ADHD have not worked, get your child comprehensively re-evaluated by a specialist to revisit the diagnosis, to rule out any other psychiatric condition (attention may be affected as a result of depression, anxiety disorders, OCD, post-traumatic stress disorder, and other conditions) or a medical condition (hypothyroidism, neurological, vision or auditory difficulties or others) or a learning disorder, all of which are known to cause attention problems. Sometimes, if the above is not helpful, neuropsychological testing can shed more light. In addition, with the help of your child's psychiatrist, attempt again to gain a deeper understanding of your child's school, social and inner life, to explore any stressors or factors that might be contributing to inattention.

31. My child is not gaining weight at all, although stimulant medicines are working well for his ADHD. What are the options?

In general, if a child is having difficulty gaining weight while taking stimulant medications, the pediatrician will closely monitor the child's growth using a growth chart and may recommend a nutritional supplement.

Other strategies such as, timing the stimulant medication after breakfast and/or allowing after-dinner snacks (when the stimulant has worn off) may allow the child to catch up on food intake. However, if the child's growth still remains significantly below the normal percentile range, and assuming it is determined that your child needs ADHD medication, the pediatrician may consider alternate medication options for your child, such as non-stimulant medications.

32. What are some behavioral Interventions for ADHD?

Even though medications are considered first line for most cases of ADHD, behavioral interventions are imperative for children with ADHD. Without school-based interventions and a clear behavioral strategy at home, ADHD management may not be optimal.

For young children age 4-5 years, the American Academy of Pediatrics has recommended behavior therapy as the first line treatment for ADHD. Behavior therapy usually involves a behavioral plan (based on age appropriate rewards, token economy, structure, consistent/firm limits) and parent behavior modification training.

Following are some behavioral strategies:

a) *Feedback:*

A high ratio of positive to constructive feedback is very important for your

ADHD child/teen. Children and teens with ADHD often receive a high degree of negative feedback at home as well as at school. This can predispose them to developing low self- esteem, depression, getting bullied or even bullying others.

b) *Pick your battles:*

Criticizing every annoying behavior that your ADHD child/teen engages in, will only serve them to tune you out eventually. Instead, in order to be effective, *praise desirable behavior in a specific manner* (saying 'good job' is good, but, not enough. Describe the behavior more specifically as well as reward/praise it right away, when feasible).

c) *Consequences, rewards:*

Prolonged time-outs or prolonged withdrawal of privileges tends to feel punitive to a child or teen. Make the consequences and rewards immediate, or as close to the behavior as feasible. A reward that occurs 7 days from the time of the actual desirable behavior will not link the behavior with the reward for your child.

d) *Structure, limits:*

Firm, consistent (while empathic) limits and structure can greatly help children and teens with ADHD.

e) *Social skills training*, individual or group:

This can assist with social difficulties that children with ADHD may experience. Your child's school may have a social skills group. If not, your physician may be able to refer to such a group in the area.

Sleep Difficulty

Sleep is one of the most important basic physiological functions. There is no replacement or substitute for it. However, millions of people across the world suffer from difficulty falling and/or staying asleep, or unrestful sleep.

The following hypothetical questions and answers are aimed at shedding light on some causes of sleep difficulty and effective treatment strategies.

33.My husband snores loudly at night. He has been receiving treatment for depression for years, which has helped a lot. Sleep medication helps him fall asleep, but, he still feels like he hasn't slept well. He dozes off during the day while watching TV or reading. I am at a loss about his sleep issues.

A physician/sleep specialist can help uncover the cause and recommend suitable treatment for sleep problems. In general, in depressed individuals who snore, obstructive sleep apnea is a possibility. Depression increases risk of obstructive sleep apnea, and vice versa. In addition, individuals who are overweight/obese or have a high neck volume are at greater risk for obstructive sleep apnea.

Obstructive sleep apnea is a condition in which there are multiple interruptions of breathing per hour. Due to these interruptions, there is fragmentation of sleep and thus, poor quality sleep. In severe cases of obstructive sleep apnea, there is even risk of cardiac arrest and stroke, due to reduced blood supply to various organs as a result of interrupted breathing.

Diagnosis of obstructive sleep apnea is made by doing an overnight sleep study. This is a painless test.

Effective treatment for obstructive sleep apnea is available, and therefore, recognition of this condition is key. The cornerstone of treatment is continuous positive airway pressure (CPAP). Weight reduction, if overweight/obese, is beneficial as well.

A sleep specialist will do a thorough evaluation first and rule out other conditions which could cause similar symptoms. Understanding the root cause when feasible, and addressing it is of utmost importance.

34.I have had difficulty falling asleep for several years. What might be causing it?

If you have been suffering from difficulty falling asleep for several years, you need a comprehensive evaluation by a sleep specialist as well as your primary care physician to explore and rule out potential underlying conditions and develop a treatment plan accordingly. The physician will explore the underlying cause, so that treatment addresses the cause rather than just addressing the symptoms or acting as a band-aid.

The causes of difficulty falling asleep or initial insomnia can be many and varied, ranging from medical causes (such as, restless legs syndrome) to psychiatric causes such as anxiety or depressive disorders. Also, insomnia can sometimes be the result of a primary sleep disorder or even due to an inconsistent sleep schedule or poor sleep hygiene. Certain medications, caffeine can increase risk of insomnia.

Chronic sleep difficulty can cause difficulty focusing, memory problems, depletion of daytime energy and productivity, as well as increased risk of motor vehicle accidents. In addition, sleep difficulty can lead to harmful physiological changes by altering the levels of stress hormone.

Also see the list of sleep hygiene measures (discussed in the answer to the next question) that can help improve sleep.

35.I haven't been able to sleep well for many years. I have trouble feeling rested when I wake up. My sleep medicine helped initially, but, does not help anymore. What might be going on?

If sleep difficulty is not resolving despite months of sleep medication use, talk to your primary care doctor to explore the option of seeing a sleep specialist.

In general, sleep difficulty can be caused by a primary sleep disorder, or at times, it is secondary to a psychiatric condition (such as an anxiety disorder or depression). At times, the sleep difficulty can be due to a medical problem or due to a medication. Treatment of the underlying condition will likely ameliorate the sleep problem.

A psychiatric condition and a primary sleep disorder can even co-exist. For example, an individual may suffer from depression as well as obstructive sleep apnea. An assumption that the sleep problem is due to or only due to depression may be problematic in such a case, if the diagnosis and treatment of the underlying sleep disorder (in this case obstructive sleep apnea) get missed.

Sleep medications are typically not meant for long-term use, except in certain situations. They do not cure the underlying condition. They serve more for rapid relief of symptoms for short periods, which means that it is still important to get a thorough assessment to find out what's going on underneath that's causing your sleep problem.

After use of sleep medications for several months, you may feel like the medication is no longer working. This is because many sleep medicines work on receptors in the brain that may be linked to dependence and tolerance. This means that over time, your body may get used to it and you may need higher doses to achieve the same effect. Some sleep medications, such as trazodone, are not known to cause dependence, and thus, may be preferred for certain kinds of sleep difficulty.

Each sleep medication is different in regards to how long it lasts in your body, how long it takes to start working, and therefore, you need to share the details of your specific sleep difficulty with your doctor so that they can arrive to the correct diagnosis and recommend the most suitable treatment.

Often, sleep difficulty may improve or even resolve with proper sleep hygiene measures, especially if the sleep difficulty resulted from poor sleep hygiene. Sleep hygiene measures include simple, yet, important interventions such as:

- having a regular bedtime,
- avoiding bright light in the 2-3 hours preceding sleep,
- avoiding caffeinated drinks especially later in the day,
- keeping room temperature

comfortable,
- using bed only for sleep,
- avoiding technology use 1-2 hours prior to bedtime,
- moderate, daily physical exercise (as permitted by your primary care physician), but, preferably prior to 6 pm.

If you are having difficulty sleeping due to difficulty relaxing after a busy, hectic day, use of breathing exercises, guided meditation, visual imagery, progressive muscle relaxation techniques can help. A therapist can help with these techniques. CBT or Cognitive behavioral Therapy for Insomnia has also been proven to be effective for sleep problems that are not secondary to a medical or a primary sleep disorder.

36. I was taking 'Ambien' 5 mg nightly; it was working great, but, then, it stopped working. I am thinking of increasing the dose to 15 mg daily. I've not had any side effects from it, so, it can't hurt. Right?

One should not change doses of medications without consulting the prescribing doctor, so, talk to your doctor about it. Seemingly minor or innocuous-looking dose changes can make a huge difference in your safety and health. In this example, Zolpidem (also known by brand name, Ambien) is accompanied with a black box warning by the FDA that the dose of this medication for women be lowered from 10 mg to 5 mg daily, as women have a lower ability to eliminate this medication from their bodies. The FDA warning also highlighted that zolpidem and similar sleep medications can impair alertness and increase risk for adverse sleep related behaviors (sleep walking, sleep driving, etc.) with effects lasting even the next day. In general, people taking benzodiazepines, other sedative-hypnotics or any sleep agent, must exercise caution with driving or operating heavy machinery the next day, because these medications have the potential to cause persisting drowsiness, impaired alertness even when you think you are awake and functioning fine. It is also worth exploring and addressing other potential factors contributing to poor sleep, such as anxiety/depression or another psychiatric condition, or a primary sleep disorder such as sleep apnea (see a sleep specialist for assessment for sleep apnea). Also, sleep hygiene measures, such as having a regular bedtime, soft lights in the evening, no electronic use 1-2 hours prior to bedtime, restriction of caffeine and caffeinated drinks, exercising daily (prior to 6 or 7pm), using the bed only for sleep, ensuring a comfortable temperature in bedroom, can go a long way in promoting better sleep.

Eating Disorders

Eating disorders are debilitating conditions that can have serious physical and psychological complications. If untreated, a type of eating disorder known as anorexia, has the highest rate of mortality among all psychiatric disorders. Timely identification and treatment is crucial. Often, individuals with eating disorders develop depressive and anxiety disorders in addition. Effective treatment is available, and usually delivered via a team-based approach to ensure optimal treatment outcomes and to ensure that medical, psychiatric, social, and family based aspects of the condition are being addressed. The role of the family can be key, as individuals themselves may hide or not recognize the disorder, especially initially.

37. What does an eating disorder look like?

Eating disorders can be of three types- anorexia nervosa, bulimia and binge eating disorder. Each of these disorders presents differently, although there is some overlap.
Individuals with anorexia are significantly underweight and may miss their periods for more than 3 months consecutively. Anorexia involves food restriction/excessive dieting, may involve excessive exercising, and/or even purging in the form of forced vomiting/use of laxatives/other agents to lose weight. You don't have to have all of the above symptoms to have anorexia.

On the other hand, individuals with bulimia are more likely to have average body weight. Purging behaviors are particularly common in bulimia and may cause problems of the salivary glands (parotid glands). In severe cases, they may even cause esophageal tears, due to the effects of forced vomiting.

Eating disorders are much more common in females, although in 1% of cases, these disorders affect males.

Untreated eating disorders affect the sodium, potassium and chloride balance of the body, which in turn, increases risk of life-threatening cardiac problems. That is why, a physician may do an EKG at baseline and on a periodic basis, if they suspect an individual to be suffering from an eating disorder.

In severe cases, osteoporosis may result from loss of bone density. This is an irreversible complication of eating disorders. Consulting a physician is very important if you or a family member experiences concerns about the possibility of an eating disorder.

38. **My sister has gotten thinner and thinner over the last year. She keeps insisting that she is very fat, although most people would call her very skinny. I think she has an eating disorder. What can be done for it?**

If suspecting an eating disorder, seek the consultation and opinion of a physician for an expert recommendation. Eating disorders are serious conditions that can jeopardize the mental as well as physical health of an individual, and in rare cases, can even be life-threatening if untreated. Therefore, treatment and early recognition is of utmost importance. A physician would do a thorough and comprehensive assessment (including, but not limited to, lab testing) to rule out any other medical or psychiatric condition that may be presenting in this manner.

Individuals with eating disorders often have shame about their body and eating habits, so, they may be in denial of the severity or extent of the problem.

Gently express your concern to the affected individual and reiterate that you are there for their support while giving them more information/resources when feasible.

The good news is that eating disorder treatment has been shown to be effective and can be life-saving. It involves psychotherapy in the form of CBT (cognitive behavioral therapy), and often use of medications such as SSRIs (selective serotonin re-uptake inhibitors) besides nutritional measures for weight restoration (which is the priority, especially in severe cases). Occasionally, other medications such as atypical antipsychotics may be offered for short periods in severe cases. Treatment may be offered in outpatient or inpatient (admitted to a hospital) settings, depending on how severe the eating disorder is.

Treatment is provided usually by a team, involving an internal medicine doctor/pediatrician, a psychiatrist, a nutritionist, a psychologist/therapist, social worker, and sometimes, other specialists such as cardiologists, if needed. Family therapy based interventions are often incorporated in treatment, especially for younger individuals.

Some resources for Eating Disorders:

Eating Disorder Hope

https://www.eatingdisorderhope.com/

Gurze/Salucore Eating Disorders Resource Catalogue

https://www.edcatalogue.com/

Eating Disorder Referral and Information Center

www.edreferral.com

Anxiety Disorders, Obsessive Compulsive Disorder (OCD) and Post-Traumatic Stress Disorder

Anxiety disorders are the most common psychiatric conditions across the world. Almost 1 in 5 people in the United States suffer from an anxiety disorder. Generalized anxiety disorder, panic disorder, social phobia, specific phobias are some types of anxiety disorders. Anxiety disorders typically respond well to treatment by psychotherapy and/or medications. Benefits from psychotherapy for anxiety disorders have been shown to last even years after stopping the therapy. CBT, psychodynamic psychotherapy and other therapy approaches can be effective.

Post-traumatic stress disorder is a condition that develops in response to a traumatic event, commonly experienced by war veterans, victims of abuse. Effective treatment usually involves psychotherapy and/or medications.

39. What is anxiety? Is it always a disorder?

Anxiety is a normal evolutionary reaction to perceived dangers or threat, but, when anxiety becomes excessive, uncontrolled or exaggerated on a frequent basis, then, it can start impairing the functioning of the individual and takes the form of a disorder.

Anxiety disorders are the most common psychiatric disorders. When severe, anxiety disorders can be paralyzing-people suffering from severe anxiety disorders may excessively avoid triggering situations, sometimes for years.

Anxiety disorders can go hand in hand with depressive disorders- it is not uncommon for them to co-exist. One can often lead to the other.

In order to diagnose an anxiety disorder, the first step is an evaluation by a physician to rule out an underlying medical condition. Certain medical conditions, such as hyperthyroidism, pheochromocytoma, cardiac and lung diseases can mimic symptoms of anxiety disorders or cause anxiety. Only if it cannot be explained by a medical condition or by use of medications or substances, is an anxiety disorder considered psychiatric.

40. **My daughter suffers from generalized anxiety disorder. I give her a lot of reassurance and have agreed to her request that she need not go to school since her anxiety is so bad. However, she keeps getting more anxious and has started avoiding getting out of the house completely. Have I been approaching her anxiety the right way?**

An experienced therapist or psychiatrist can build a thoughtful, specific and tailored plan with you on how to approach your daughter's anxiety through appropriate interventions. In general, generalized anxiety has been shown to worsen in the long-term with excessive accommodations and reassurance, even though reassurance may seem to grant immediate relief to the individual.

Accommodating the avoidance that is a result of anxiety serves to fuel further avoidance of anxiety provoking situations.

The therapist/psychiatrist may also be able to work with the school counselor/special education department to develop a plan that takes into consideration the anxiety, while not reinforcing it further and also helping the child realize their optimal academic potential.

Anxiety that is severely impairing a child (or adult)'s day to day functioning typically benefits from SSRI/SNRI based medications in addition to psychotherapy. A physician/ psychiatrist will work with you to find the most suitable treatment options.

41. **I suffer from generalized anxiety disorder and panic disorder. I take my medications. I also drink a pot of coffee a day. Recently, I've noticed I'm jittery and not able to focus.**

Present your concerns to your physician. Your physician/psychiatrist will make an assessment and guide you about the next steps.
In general, there are many causes of difficulty focusing. If you have an inadequately treated/uncontrolled anxiety disorder, difficulty focusing can be a result of that. Also, caffeine is a known inducer of increased anxiety and panic attacks. That means, if you drink large amounts of coffee on a frequent basis, you are increasing your likelihood of experiencing greater anxiety and thereby, more difficulty focusing.

Inadequately controlled anxiety and depressive disorders commonly cause difficulty focusing so do ADHD (attention deficit hyperactivity disorder) and several medical conditions (such as hypothyroidism). It is important to get a thorough assessment to find out the actual cause of your difficulty focusing.

Remember that psychotherapy has been proven to have long-term benefit for anxiety and panic symptoms. Make sure the treatment for anxiety involves psychotherapy.

42. My son started taking fluoxetine for anxiety. He has been acting more anxious recently. How is that?

Consult your child's physician so that they can make an assessment and recommendations accordingly.
In general, SSRIs, such as fluoxetine, can occasionally increase anxiety (often in the short-term), especially in individuals who are already anxious, with faster dose increase, in the early phase of initiating the medication, or in the early phase of increasing the dose.

Also, some people are slow metabolizers of medications which means that they may retain the same dose of a medication to a higher level in their body than someone else, thereby, increasing risk of anxiety for them even at relatively low dosages.

For treatment of anxiety, in general, it is recommended that an SSRI be started at a low dose and increased gradually for optimal effect as tolerated.

In general, SSRIs have been shown to be effective and well-tolerated when used for various anxiety disorders.

It is also possible that the child is experiencing an increase in anxiety for reasons other than related to SSRIs. School/academic/social stressors, bullying/abuse, family stressors can be some of the reasons for increased anxiety. As always, lab testing and a medical work-up to rule out any underlying medical causes (such as hyperthyroidism) are important.

43. My child has started showing signs of obsessive compulsive disorder. He is only 9 years old, but, he repeatedly checks his school bag to make sure he has submitted his homework. He writes and re-writes his homework several times until he can get it perfect. I don't want to put him on any meds right now. Is there therapy that might work for him?

After evaluating your child, a psychiatrist will guide you about treatment options that may be most suited for your child's condition.

In general, it would be very beneficial and important for any child suspected to have OCD or another psychiatric condition, to get an evaluation by a psychiatrist or a child and adolescent psychiatrist. This helps to fully understand the child's biological, social and psychological history, stressors and triggers and to make a nuanced and effective treatment plan accordingly.

Exposure and Response Prevention (ERP) therapy is a branch of CBT (Cognitive behavioral therapy). ERP is considered to be the gold standard treatment for obsessive compulsive disorder, and is known to be effective by itself for mild to moderate obsessive compulsive disorder in children, adolescents and adults. For severe symptoms, guidelines recommend a combination of ERP and medication treatment (typically SSRIs, or clomipramine).

44. My husband likes everything very clean. I think he has OCD.

Help your husband consult a physician for a complete evaluation for an accurate diagnosis and treatment.

In general, someone who likes 'everything clean' may have OCD (Obsessive Compulsive Disorder) or another condition, or they may simply like cleanliness. The desire for cleanliness, like many other traits, lies on a spectrum. People may be on different ends of the spectrum and still fall within the normal range.

In order to meet criteria for OCD, one has to experience obsessive thoughts or compulsive behaviors for at least 1 hour a day, for 6 months or more, and the symptoms must be significantly impairing daily functioning in one or more life domains (social, work, school, etc.), according to criteria by the Diagnostic and Statistical Manual of Psychiatry (DSM-5). The symptoms should not be explained by another psychiatric, or medical condition.

If found to have OCD, there are evidence-based treatments, such as SSRI based medications, Exposure and Response Prevention therapy, which have been found to be effective for OCD. A psychiatrist evaluates and treats OCD.

45. I have been diagnosed with post-traumatic stress disorder. I've been asking my psychiatrist to prescribe me 'ativan' (generic name, lorazepam) for my feelings of anxiety. He's refusing to prescribe that. Why is that?

There could be many reasons as to why your psychiatrist is refusing to prescribe lorazepam or other benzodiazepine medications for your condition. One of them may be that research evidence shows that benzodiazepines (such as lorazepam) are not effective or recommended for PTSD and may even have negative effects for people suffering from PTSD.

In general, benzodiazepines are typically and mostly recommended for short-term use for anxiety or insomnia, often in crisis situations. They provide rapid symptom relief in the immediate, short-term, but, may not do much to address the underlying cause or the disorder itself. However, there may be certain exceptions where some people may need benzodiazepines for longer, but, that is a specific determination made by a psychiatrist who has evaluated and monitored the individual's condition for a while.

Note: Benzodiazepines should not be stopped suddenly as sudden discontinuation can lead to withdrawal symptoms, including but not limited to, insomnia, increased anxiety, risk of seizures. Instead of stopping abruptly, in most cases, benzodiazepines are usually tapered over time, on a step-by-step basis, as advised by and under the monitoring of a physician. This is especially important if you have been taking benzodiazepines for some time. Other examples of benzodiazepines are alprazolam (known more commonly by brand name, Xanax), clonazepam, diazepam (known more commonly by brand name, Valium).

Bipolar Disorder

Bipolar disorder is a type of mood disorder. It involves episodes of mania, hypomania, depression and at times, mixed episodes. At times, it can involve psychotic symptoms-these typically require hospitalization. If untreated, it can result in dangerous or risky behavior and related complications, substance and alcohol use, increased risk of suicide, and a decline in functioning. Bipolar disorder has a strong biological basis. Having a family member with bipolar disorder can increase risk of having bipolar. Medications are effective and an essential crux of treatment.

Several medications have been scientifically tested, approved and widely used for bipolar disorder. In addition to medications, being aware of triggers for these episodes is also helpful in preventing them. Maintaining adequate sleep is crucial.

46.I have bipolar disorder; I was feeling great, so, I stopped taking my medications. Is that okay?

One should not start or stop taking psychotropic medications without consulting the prescribing physician. Many medications have discontinuation or withdrawal effects if you stop taking them abruptly. Not only that, you are at risk for relapse or worsening of your psychiatric condition, if you stop your medications abruptly without talking with your doctor.

Bipolar disorder usually requires maintenance medications to prevent relapse of manic, hypomanic or depressive episodes. Many individuals with bipolar disorder make the mistake of stopping their medications when they feel good, only to have another manic or hypomanic episode. Scientific evidence shows that the more number of manic, hypomanic or depressive episodes an individual with bipolar disorder has, the more the likelihood of increased frequency and worsened course of the mood episodes. That is why, timely treatment and continued monitoring is important.

Mood stabilizers or atypical antipsychotic medications are commonly used for the treatment of bipolar disorder. Examples of mood stabilizers are lithium, valproate, lamotrigine, carbamazepine, oxcarbazepine. Examples of atypical antipsychotic medications are aripiprazole, risperidone, quetiapine, olanzapine. Use of these medications requires regular monitoring by a physician. Medications for bipolar disorder can be very effective in resolving symptoms.

47. My boyfriend has ups and downs in mood. I think he has bipolar. Is that correct?

Do not self-diagnose. Seek the consultation of a licensed physician or a licensed mental health professional for a diagnostic opinion.

While bipolar disorder presents with significant mood changes, having mood ups and downs by itself usually does not qualify for bipolar disorder. Mood changes can be due to a depressive disorder, adjustment disorder, post-traumatic stress disorder, intermittent explosive disorder, bipolar disorder, personality disorder or may even represent an underlying medical condition. The mood changes in each of these conditions may be somewhat different and require expert and nuanced assessment by a psychiatrist, psychologist or licensed mental health clinician.

Bipolar disorder is present in 1-2% of the population. Mood changes in bipolar disorder are usually a distinct change from baseline and are episodic. They are accompanied by a decreased need for sleep, with a marked increase in energy during these periods, besides other symptoms such as hypersexuality, impulsivity, and/or pressured speech during these periods. Your friends or family can usually sense that you are not acting like your usual self during these episodes- this is true even for a hypomanic episode which is less severe as compared to a manic episode.

Psychotic Disorders

Psychotic disorders are serious conditions that involve anomalies in thoughts and reality testing. Examples of psychotic disorders that are due to a psychiatric condition, are schizophrenia, schizoaffective disorder.

Sometimes, medical problems, such as a tumor or an infection in the brain can cause psychotic symptoms. Use of alcohol, cocaine, methamphetamines and other substances can cause psychotic symptoms, during states of withdrawal/intoxication. Rarely, certain medications can cause psychotic symptoms. Addressing the cause is important.

Many scientific studies have shown efficacy of treatments for psychotic disorders. Timely diagnosis and treatment is important.

48. What is a delusion? What is usually not a delusion?

A delusion is a false, fixed belief. A delusion may be bizarre or non-bizarre. Delusions can be of varied kinds, such as delusion of grandiosity, infidelity, persecutory, somatic or other.
The term delusion is often used loosely. However, 'delusion' is a specific clinical entity.

A delusion is different from an overvalued idea which is a false belief that is not held with the same degree of rigidity as a delusion. An individual holding an overvalued idea is more open to reasoning, questioning or entertaining the notion that the belief may not be accurate or true, as compared to an individual with a delusion.

A belief that is typically held by or falls within the normal range of an individual's culture is not a delusion, even though the belief may seem bizarre to people outside of that culture.

49. What are signs and symptoms of Schizophrenia?

If you are concerned about the possibility of schizophrenia, consult a physician/psychiatrist for a complete evaluation.

Symptoms of schizophrenia may be delusions, paranoia, hallucinations (commonly in the form of 'voices'), disorganized speech, or disorganized behavior. Many people with schizophrenia suffer from depressive symptoms, social withdrawal, and cognitive difficulties as well. Not all of these symptoms need to be present for a diagnosis of schizophrenia.

Example of Distorted Reality Testing:

For instance, an individual suffering from schizophrenia may believe that he/she is living on the planet Venus and be out of touch with reality.

Example of Delusions:

An individual may hold a false, fixed belief that people are organizing to persecute her/him, or that there are insects crawling on the individual's skin, even when no evidence for any of this exists. Delusions can be of many other types.

Example of Hallucinations:

Hallucinations in schizophrenia are commonly auditory. An individual affected with hallucinations may appear to be talking to people who are not there or may hear voices talking to him/her (or voices talking to each other), that nobody else can hear.

A psychiatrist can diagnose and treat schizophrenia. Effective treatments are available.

50. What is the treatment for schizophrenia?

If you or your family member suffers from schizophrenia or another primary psychotic disorder, your psychiatrist or physician will work closely with you to find a medication and dose that is most suited for your body and condition. In general, antipsychotic medications are the cornerstone of treatment for schizophrenia. Supportive and other psychotherapy can help manage stressors as well as depressive and anxiety symptoms related to the illness, however, medications are key, especially if active psychotic symptoms are present.

With adequate treatment, outreach and community support, many individuals with schizophrenia can have a decent level of functioning.

Antipsychotic medications tend to be very effective and can be life-changing in resolving the psychotic symptoms of schizophrenia. They fall into two broad categories- older or typical antipsychotics and newer or atypical antipsychotics.

Antipsychotic medications help to regulate the dopamine level in the brain, thereby, facilitating remission of psychotic symptoms. Newer antipsychotics, also known as atypical antipsychotics, are aripiprazole, olanzapine, quetiapine, risperidone, ziprasidone, lurasidone and others. Many of these antipsychotic medications are available in monthly or biweekly long-acting injectable formulations, which can make it easier to have good symptom control without having to remember to take pills every day.

Family education and support (particularly through organizations such as NAMI) can play a vital role in treatment as well.

Miscellaneous

51.My mother is in her late 80s. Recently, she developed a urinary tract infection, and since then, she has been acting weird. I'm not sure if she took the antibiotics for her UTI or not, but, she seems confused at times and seems to get agitated without any reason. This is not like her. What might be going on?

Any time there is a sudden/recent and significant change in an individual's behavior or personality, particularly in the elderly, it warrants immediate medical attention.

In general, UTIs, other medical conditions and use of certain medications can occasionally result in delirium, especially in the elderly. Delirium is a serious medical condition which can be life-threatening if untreated, and therefore, warrants emergency medical attention by taking the individual to the ER or calling 911. An emergency room physician will do a comprehensive assessment and may admit the individual for further evaluation and intensive treatment.

An individual with delirium may appear confused, agitated (or overly quiet on the other hand), may see things that others can't see (visual hallucinations), or experience other changes in their cognition.

The causes of delirium can be many and varied. The most important aspect of delirium treatment is to find and treat the underlying cause. Talk to your doctor for any concerns.

52. I am experiencing some sexual side effects from Zoloft, but, otherwise, it is working well for me. What are my options?

In general, sexual side effects are common with SSRIs (including sertraline- brand name, Zoloft). These side effects are typically reversible when medication is stopped. Sexual side effects can occur in the form of delayed ejaculation/orgasm, decreased libido. For an individual experiencing sexual side effects after the start of SSRIs, the psychiatrist may discuss the option of lowering the SSRI. Sometimes, these side effects go away at a reduced dose while efficacy of the medication can still be maintained.

Alternatively, the doctor may discuss lowering the dose of SSRI and/or adding a medication such as bupropion (an antidepressant which acts on different receptors such as dopamine) to counter the sexual side effects. There are other medication options as well that can help mitigate sexual side effects from SSRIs. Your physician will help determine if you need one.

Other antidepressant medications, such as SNRIs, and older antidepressants (such as tricyclic antidepressants), can also cause sexual side effects.

However, not everyone who takes these medications will experience such side effects.

53. Will I get dependent on this medication once I start taking it?

Always ask your doctor if you have any questions about medications or treatment. In general, there are certain medications which can create dependence.
These are controlled substances (for example, benzodiazepines, certain sleep agents) which have varying degree of potential for dependence. They work on certain receptors in the brain which are linked with dependence. Therefore, use of such medications should be only under the regular monitoring of a doctor. Other commonly used psychotropic medications, such as antidepressants (SSRIs, SNRIs or others), mood stabilizers, and antipsychotics do not cause dependence.

For this reason, FDA has recommended that use of benzodiazepines should be time limited. However, benzodiazepines should not be stopped abruptly as they can cause withdrawal symptoms such as seizures, increase in anxiety or insomnia with sudden discontinuation. Your doctor will advise you on when and how to gradually taper off your medication if you determine together that you need to.

54. My pupils seem bigger. I haven't changed anything, except that the dose of my venlafaxine was raised a week ago. Could it have something to do with that?

If you have new/sudden difficulty with bright light and/or someone tells you your pupils seem bigger, you should contact your doctor immediately, so that they can advise you about the next best course of action.

In general, venlafaxine, which is an SNRI, can occasionally cause pupil dilation. Dose decrease usually relieves this side effect. In some cases, stopping the medication may be necessary. In general, if any medication side effect is severe/rapidly worsening, you should seek emergency medical attention by going to the emergency room or calling 911 and providing the doctor with a complete list of your medications along with a history of any changes, recent travel, insect bites or other exposures.

55. I have been taking haloperidol for more than 2 decades for schizophrenia. Recently, my friend noticed that the area around my mouth and lip has been twitching frequently. I haven't started any new medication or changed my medication dosage recently. Could this be related to Haloperidol?

Anytime you are noticing any new/recent/worsening physical or psychological concerns, consult your physician/psychiatrist to determine the next best course of action. Haloperidol or any other antipsychotic medication has the potential to cause twitching or lip smacking movements around the mouth and lip area, when used in long-term. This is known as tardive dyskinesia. This side effect can be irreversible. However, not everyone develops it. Some people are at higher risk for it than others. Older antipsychotics (known as typical antipsychotics, such as haloperidol, fluphenazine) are more likely to cause tardive dyskinesia than newer ones (known as atypical antipsychotics, such as aripiprazole, quetiapine and others). Seeing your psychiatrist on a regular basis can help them catch early signs of tardive dyskinesia, so that together, you can consider a dose decrease or even a medication change if needed, to prevent TD. The AIMS test (Abnormal Involuntary Movement Scale) is a screening tool that your psychiatrist will use to assess for and track any abnormal movements. Sometimes, people are tempted to stop their medications on hearing about a possible side effect. Stopping medications suddenly is usually not a good idea unless the side effect you are experiencing is severe/extreme or you are stopping at the recommendation of your doctor. Sudden stoppage of medication can lead to relapse and/or withdrawal or discontinuation effects.

56. I tried taking a pill from my friend who has ….. (ADHD/anxiety/other psychiatric condition). It worked great, I want my doctor to prescribe it for me.

In general, it is not only illegal to take a medication prescribed to someone else (at least in the United States), but also, can be harmful or even life-threatening. Your friend, child, parent, sibling is not you. Each individual's biological and psychological predispositions and psychiatric condition are unique. The same medication can affect your body quite differently than it does someone else's.

Do not take medication prescribed for someone else. Consult your doctor to discuss your concerns, so that you can find a suitable treatment option tailored to your specific condition.

57. What is the difference between a psychologist and a psychiatrist? How do I know who to see?

A psychiatrist is a medical doctor, someone who has graduated from medical school and specialized (completed 4 years of residency training) in the field of psychiatry. A psychiatrist can assess, diagnose, and treat psychiatric conditions using medications, psychotherapy and/or other modalities such as ECT (Electroconvulsive Therapy), TMS (Transcranial Magnetic Stimulation), etc. Psychiatrists may refer their patients to psychologists or therapists for psychotherapy.

A psychologist is someone who has completed a PhD or a PsyD in the field of Psychology, after doing a masters in psychology. A psychologist may specialize in one or various kinds of psychotherapy treatments. In addition, psychologists may perform psychological testing, such as, dementia testing or neuropsychological testing. Barring a few states, psychologists are not licensed to prescribe or manage medications.

Psychiatrists and psychologists often work closely together to coordinate the care of a patient.

In addition, there are licensed mental health professionals such as social workers, mental health counselors, who also provide psychotherapy.

58. What does a psychiatrist do? I am hesitant to see one. I don't want people to think I am 'crazy'.

A psychiatrist is a medical doctor who specializes in the field of psychiatry. A psychiatrist can diagnose, assess and treat psychiatric conditions or disorders. Examples of psychiatric disorders are depression, anxiety disorders, bipolar disorder, obsessive compulsive disorder, schizophrenia, post-traumatic stress disorder. If you suspect your emotional/mental state is not good, you should see a psychiatrist, or discuss your symptoms with your primary doctor along with a potential referral to a psychiatrist.

A few decades ago, there was greater stigma in seeing a psychiatrist or seeking mental health treatment. Nowadays, this stigma is declining as we are getting to know not only that mental health disorders are highly prevalent, but also, that these disorders also have a biological basis and involve changes in the functioning of the brain; these are not 'character weaknesses'.

According to the World Health Organization estimates, about 1 in 4 people across the world would suffer from a psychiatric or neurological disorder at some point. This means psychiatric conditions have reached epidemic proportions. It means that one person in every family may end up suffering from a psychiatric or a neurological condition. Psychiatric conditions are treatable, and newer and more effective treatment options are being researched daily.

Untreated psychiatric conditions pose significant risk of worsening over time and have been proven by research to cause negative and detrimental brain changes.

A psychiatrist can provide treatment for these disorders by doing a comprehensive evaluation, recommending psychotherapy, and/or prescribing psychotropic medications. If your condition is severe, they may discuss other treatment options with you such as inpatient hospitalization, intensive outpatient program or others.

Whatever you discuss inside your psychiatrist's office stays confidential. Barring certain exceptions, a psychiatrist will not disclose to anyone what you reveal to them. With your consent, your psychiatrist may discuss certain details of your condition with your family, your primary care doctor and/or therapist when suitable.

Having a psychiatric condition does not mean you are 'crazy'. Psychiatric conditions are very common across the world and can affect anyone. Most importantly, there are effective treatments for psychiatric disorders; these treatments can markedly improve quality of life.

59. Medications have Side Effects! Why Would I Want to Take Them?

That's a valid question. Almost everyone taking medications has wondered about this at some point.

Just like medications for other medical conditions such as asthma, hypertension or diabetes, psychotropic medications have potential side effects as well. All medications have potential side effects; that does not mean that everyone who takes a particular medication will experience a side effect. In fact, a significant proportion of people taking a psychotropic medication will not experience any side effects at all.

The decision to take a medication is preceded by careful weighing of benefits and side effects, risks. It depends on your individual clinical condition, its severity, and its impact on your life and functioning.

Untreated psychiatric disorders (such as depression) have been shown to cause harmful structural and functional changes in the brain. If the benefit of taking a medication overweighs the risks/side-effects from that medication, and your psychiatric condition is impairing your functioning significantly, your physician/psychiatrist may recommend a psychotropic medication to you.

You should be forthcoming with your physician about any questions or concerns you may have about medications. Your physician is in the position to help you best if they really know what's going on with you.

60. Do I have to take my medications lifelong?

The answer to that depends on which psychiatric condition you are suffering from, and on the severity of your psychiatric condition. Your psychiatrist will advise you on the most appropriate approach based on the specifics of yore condition.

For example, if you've had several hospitalizations for repeated episodes of severe depression, it is likely that your doctor may recommend taking antidepressant medication long-term.

On the other hand, if you suffer from an anxiety disorder as a result of a recent job loss or other stressor and this is the first time you've suffered from significant anxiety, you may not need medications for more than a year or two if you achieve stability with treatment. The determination of when to stop medications should be made only under the consultation and monitoring of your physician or psychiatrist.

Psychotropic medications need to be monitored regularly, and the need to take them or the need for dose adjustment (increase or decrease) needs to be assessed on a regular basis by your prescribing doctor. Feel free to bring forth your questions to your doctor so that your doctor can help you make informed decisions for the best treatment outcomes.

61. My girlfriend is a counselor, so, I don't need a therapist. She can help me. Is that right?

Having a family member or a loved one who is in the mental health field, can be very helpful. This family member/loved one/friend can guide you towards the right resources and can help you navigate new and complex systems. However, family members or friends cannot serve as your therapist.

Part of what makes therapy effective is that a therapist is able to be objective and professional. A family member/friend is likely to be emotionally invested in you, have his/her own biases, and for several reasons, would not be the right person to be your therapist.

62. How do I find a therapist or a psychiatrist? I don't know how to go about it.

There are a few ways to find a therapist or a psychiatrist:

- Your primary care physician/family physician/pediatrician may be able to refer you to a therapist or a psychiatrist.

- You can find a therapist through this link: https://www.psychologytoday.com/us/therapists

- You can find a psychiatrist through this link: http://finder.psychiatry.org/

- You should be able to find a list of local therapists or psychiatrists covered by your insurance, by calling your insurance company.

63. I tried therapy for a little bit, but, didn't feel like me and my therapist clicked. I don't see any point in going to a therapist anymore.

Sometimes, you may feel like there isn't a rapport between you and your therapist. Therapy is supposed to be a safe space; feel free to share with your therapist what about the therapy sessions is not working with you. Your therapist is not likely to be offended or judge you for that. Sometimes, what's not working out in therapy may shed light on other underlying themes or patterns in your life, which may be beneficial for you and your therapist to explore and understand together.

Psychotherapy can be transformational and life-changing. Evidence from scientific studies shows that the benefits of good, evidence-based psychotherapy can last for years after the therapy is stopped.

If you still feel like this particular therapist's style is really not working, or not a good fit for you, do not give up. Find another therapist who may be more suitable for you.

Feel free to ask questions, such as what kind of therapy the therapist specializes in, what their area of expertise is, what age group they commonly see, etcetera, when looking for therapists.

64. Will my insurance cover me seeing a therapist and a psychiatrist?

Most insurances cover seeing a psychiatrist and a therapist for most psychiatric disorders. You can call your insurance to find out specifically what mental health benefits are covered by your insurance. It is possible that your insurance covers certain therapists and psychiatrists in your area and doesn't cover others. In addition, some therapists and psychiatrists are able to see patients on a sliding scale fee basis.

The American Psychiatric Association and other associations have been advocating for mental health benefits to be covered at the same level as benefits for medical conditions.

65. What are the different kinds of psychotherapy approaches?

There are various modalities of psychotherapy treatments that are evidence based and proven to be effective.
Here are some commonly used types of psychotherapies:

Psychodynamic Psychotherapy:

The oldest form of psychotherapy is psychoanalysis, which is utilized less commonly nowadays. A modified offshoot of psychoanalysis is psychodynamic psychotherapy, which aims to address a condition by exploring, uncovering and understanding underlying unconscious conflicts that may be rooted often in the developmental period. This kind of psychotherapy is effective for personality disorders, depressive, anxiety and some other psychiatric disorders. An individual who is: motivated for change, able to bear the frustration that can come out of digging deep into one's own personality and relational patterns, and who is not currently going through an acute crisis, may be a good candidate for undergoing this type of psychotherapy.

Psychodynamic psychotherapy typically runs longer as compared to cognitive behavioral therapy, dialectical behavior therapy or other newer therapies. Mostly due to this reason and because newer, manualized forms of psychotherapy have been researched to a greater extent, the newer psychotherapy approaches are utilized more commonly these days. Psychodynamic psychotherapy is offered by a relatively smaller percentage of psychotherapists and psychiatrists nowadays, even though it is effective. Brief psychodynamic psychotherapy is a type of psychodynamic psychotherapy that is focused on addressing a specific problem and is of shorter duration.

CBT (Cognitive Behavioral Therapy):

Cognitive behavioral therapy or CBT is a commonly used form of psychotherapy that has been studied extensively in the last few decades. CBT helps the affected individual identify and challenge maladaptive thoughts and beliefs. With the help of CBT, distorted beliefs linked to certain thoughts or mood are identified and changed. CBT typically requires 12-16 sessions. CBT is effective for anxiety disorders, depressive disorders, eating disorders, and other psychiatric conditions. CBT is also effective for insomnia.

Interpersonal Therapy:

Interpersonal therapy usually involves 12-16 sessions, and is beneficial for grief or loss, role transitions (related to illness or other life events). The therapist helps facilitate the individual's coping with and understanding of a particular life change/event or stressor.

DBT (Dialectical Behavioral Therapy):

This form of psychotherapy developed as a branch of CBT and is now commonly used. It incorporates mindfulness techniques for distress tolerance and emotional regulation. It can be especially effective for individuals suffering from repeated self-injurious thoughts or behavior. It is also considered an effective form of therapy for individuals suffering from borderline personality disorder.

In addition to the above, there are also other kinds of psychotherapies, such as mindfulness-based stress reduction, rational emotive therapy and others.

Psychotherapy may be offered in individual, group or couples settings, depending on the clinical situation.

References

American Academy of Child and Adolescent Psychiatry. Facts for Families Guide. Depression in Children and Teens. Retrieved April 8, 2018, from https://www.aacap.org/AACAP/Families_and_youth/Facts_for_Families/FFF-Guide/The-Depressed-Child-004.aspx

American Academy of Family Physicians (AAFP). Retrieved April 8, 2018, from https://www.aafp.org/patient-care/clinical-recommendations/all/myocardial.html

Bhatia, R. 'Rule out these Causes of Inattention before diagnosing ADHD'. Current Psychiatry, 2016 October;15(10):32-C3.

Centers for Disease Control and Prevention. Attention-Deficit/Hyperactivity Disorder (ADHD). ADHD Home: Basic Information. Retrieved April 1, 2018, from https://www.cdc.gov/ncbddd/adhd/facts.html

Centers for Disease Control and Prevention. Healthy Aging. Retrieved April 8, 2018, from https://www.cdc.gov/aging/mentalhealth/depression.htm

Desk Reference to the Diagnostic Criteria from DSM-5. American Psychiatric Association.

Mattes, JA. Treating ADHD in Prison: Focus on Alpha-2 Agonists (Clonidine and Guanfacine). The Journal of the American Academy of Psychiatry and the Law. Volume 44, Number 2, 2016.

Mayo Clinic. Patient Care and Health Information. Tests and Procedures. Light Therapy. Retrieved on April 28, 2018, from https://www.mayoclinic.org/tests-procedures/light-therapy/about/pac-20384604

MGH Center for Women's Mental Health: Reproductive Psychiatry Resource and Information Center. Psychiatric Disorders during Pregnancy. Retrieved on April 15, 2018, from

https://womensmentalhealth.org/specialty-clinics/psychiatric-disorders-during-pregnancy/

National Institute of Mental Health. Health and Education. Mental Health Information. Depression. Retrieved on April 8, 2018, from https://www.nimh.nih.gov/health/topics/depression/index.shtml

National Institute of Mental Health. Health and Education. Publications. NIMH Answers Questions About Suicide. Retrieved on April 8, 2018, from https://www.nimh.nih.gov/health/publications/nimh-answers-questions-about-suicide/index.shtml

National Institute of Mental Health. Health and Education. Mental Health Information. Brain Stimulation Therapies. Retrieved on April 8, 2018, from https://www.nimh.nih.gov/health/topics/brain-stimulation-therapies/brain-stimulation-therapies.shtml

World Health Organization (April 2017). Mental Disorders Fact Sheet. Retrieved on April 1, 2018, from http://www.who.int/mediacentre/factsheets/fs396/en/

Resources

National Institute of Mental Health. Health Information.
https://www.nimh.nih.gov/health/publications/index.shtml

Centers for Disease Prevention and Control (CDC).
https://www.cdc.gov/mentalhealth/index.htm

American Academy of Child and Adolescent Psychiatry. Facts for Families Guide.
https://www.aacap.org/AACAP/Families_and_Youth/Facts_for_Families/FFF-Guide/FFF-Guide-Home.aspx

World Health Organization. Mental Health. Mental Disorders.
http://www.who.int/mental_health/management/en/

American Foundation for Suicide Prevention.
https://afsp.org/

ABOUT THE AUTHOR

Richa Bhatia, MD is a dual Board-certified Child, Adolescent and Adult Psychiatrist, and a Fellow of the American Psychiatric Association. She has served as a Faculty Member in the departments of Psychiatry at Harvard Medical School and at Geisel School of Medicine at Dartmouth. She is the recipient of Marian Butterfield award by the Association of Women Psychiatrists. Dr. Bhatia is the Author of the book: 'Demystifying Psychiatric Conditions and Treatments, and Answers to Your Commonly Asked Questions'. She serves as the Associate Editor for Current Psychiatry and on the editorial board of other psychiatry journals. She has been invited to speak at national and international conferences.

Over the years, Dr. Bhatia has treated thousands of patients suffering from various psychiatric conditions in various clinical settings. She espouses the integration of psychotherapy and psychopharmacological approaches in treatment along with empathic, evidence-based practices.